I0430189

Forget Perfect, Just Be Better

101 Simple Ways to Be a Better Person in Your Relationships, at Work, in Life, and Through God

By Richard N. Stephenson

Table of Contents

All Rights Reserved © 2014 RichardStep.com Publishing

Perfect is Impossible

It's that day. That day when things couldn't get any worse. That day when you just want to shrink away and hide. That's the day when the little voice in your head pokes through the noise and says, "You know what? I want to be a better person. I can do more than this. I deserve more than this."

And you know what? You do! All you have to do is ask yourself when, specifically, do you want to start to change? And if you're able to ask that question, then you're capable of coming up with the answer. It's that straight-forward.

That doesn't mean change is easy. Simple, sure, but it's not easy.

When you're dirty, can you take a shower to get clean? How long does that cleanliness last? Do you need to take a shower the next day to keep the stink off? In order to stay clean and in good working order, you're going to have to do the work of showering every day. Change isn't a one-time process, it's a lifelong habit.

You can give yourself permission to change when you want to. You can do that right now. You can give yourself permission to stop trying to be perfect and instead start being a little better. Not much, just one-percent here and there. It's up to you. Aim for a little bit better than yesterday and start to notice the change in your life.

Will it take some work? Of course. Will you be lifted out of your comfort zone? Absolutely. Is this a scary thing? Maybe. Is it necessary to grow? You tell me. Does a tree grow by staying a comfortable seed? Or does it have to tear through the ground, fight bad weather, and fend off pesky birds every day of its life?

You're Ready to Be a Better You

I don't want to drag on forever convincing you how important change is and how important it is to be committed to the process of growth. I know you're capable, intelligent, and don't need to be lectured to. I know by your consideration in getting this book, you're looking for some ideas.

And that's exactly what you'll get here.

How does this book connect to your bigger picture? The examples inside are all simple and practical ways to clear out the junk in your life and make room for the good stuff. Think of this as an idea book for ways to improve your life, one manageable step at a time.

These aren't just any 101 ways to be a better person. You shouldn't try to slam through and do them all in one week. These are bite-sized chunks of challenging, useful, and practical exercises to get your mind right and your world in order. These are one-percent change ideas you can handle.

There's one main thing you need to do before you head down this change journey. You have to answer two questions for yourself:

1) What do you want your new self to look like, sound like, act like, feel like, and be like?

2) How is changing your life important to you?

Notice that question two asks why it is important to you, not anyone else. Keep your family, friends, and the world in mind, of course. But you have to know that your main focus here is to change the only thing you have control over in this whole world: you.

You can change yourself to make your life better.
You can become a better person to do more things.
You can do more things, better, to help others more.
You can help others better, to live your life more fully.
You can be a better person, when you stop trying to be perfect and just be better.

The Lifelong Journey Begins

Something that always bugged me about the personal development field was the lack of practical examples to take action on. Sure, I know I need to be a better person, but how the hee-haw am I supposed to do it, specifically? Examples - I need examples!

I couldn't find the answer to that question, so I wrote my own answers - a whopping 101 of them.

Over the following pages you will get tons of immediately usable ideas to make your life just a little bit better, one piece at a time. I cover as many bases as I can without trying to write an encyclopedia. People are complex and no two are exactly alike. The more choices we have in life, the better.

These are the areas of your life covered in this book:

*Be a Better Person At Work
*Be a Better Person In Relationships
*Be a Better Person Through God
*Be a Better Person By Being Healthy
*Be a Better Person By Learning
*Be a Better Person Through Success
*Be a Better Person Through Creativity
*Be a Better Person By Exploring
*Be a Better Person Through Thinking
*Be a Better Person By Having Fun
*Be a Better Person By Communicating
*Be a Better Person By Cleaning Chaos
*Be a Better Person In Society

Each one of the 101 ways has an actionable step for you to take to practice being a better person. These are the "Just Be Better" exercises. You can start from the beginning and work your way through, step by step, or you can open this book at a random location and pick one.

The key is to get in the habit of looking. Find something you want to try, give it an honest, open, and true effort, and see what you learn. The worst that could happen is you learn only a little. The best that could happen is that you learn a whole dang lot.

There's no way you can lose here. You're safe. You're safe to give these ideas your best shot and see what comes out. I know you can do it because I've done it. If I can do it, you can do it. These aren't empty promises - these are facts, my friend.

Suspend your disbeliefs, your critiques, and your doubts for a while and have a dang good time making your life better, one-percent at a time.

Forget Perfect, Just Be Better.

*****

Be A Better Person:

AT WORK

A lot of us hold our careers very near and dear to our hearts. Does this mean we absolutely love them to death? Maybe, maybe not. But it does mean something that happens at work directly impacts our mood, our income, and our families. That's a big deal. Let's get our work life in shape to let the good feelings funnel down and around to the other parts of our life.

1) Be Great to Your Cube Mate

When I'm at work, I like to be busy doing stuff that makes a difference. But every once in a while I'm pushing so hard I lose my super-cheery attitude and go into "gotta get it done" mode. It's usually about this time someone slips a candy or two onto my desk without my knowing. Such a nice little surprise and it helps anchor me back to my good place. Much appreciated.

We can sometimes fall into the trap of forgetting we're working with people, and not just coworkers. If you constantly think of Bobby Joe as "just the guy who packages stuff," then you're doing a real disservice to yourself, Bobby Joe, and the company. We need to remind ourselves to step back every once in a while, realize that we're dealing with honest-to-goodness people, and work will get done better if we work everything out.

Just Be Better: Ask other people if they need help with something today. If they say no, gently press a little bit and see what you can help out with. If they offer a choice, don't pick the easiest choice. Heck, go buy them a fancy coffee or refreshing tea as an added surprise.

Be a cubical ninja of kindness.

2) Inbox: Ground Zero

Too many times I've been to a meeting where the person presenting has Outlook open. In addition to the twenty-three reminders that pop up in the middle of the presentation, there are usually hundreds of unread emails glaring at them. I can't understand how anyone is encouraged to work with Outlook when this mass of time-consuming junk is always staring them in the face. That's a lot of pressure.

Anxiety, stress, and a feeling of overwhelming burden can settle in when things start to get out of control in important areas of your life. Don't think it's that big of a deal? Do you have a pile of mail sitting on a table at home? How high is it? I'm guessing it's not high at all, if it even exists. At home, it's easier to see how such a mess of "things to do" can grate on your wellbeing. Well, just because those "to do's" are digital it doesn't mean it's not affecting your mental stability in some way.

Just Be Better: Clean out your email inbox using the four level approach. (1) Do the quick stuff immediately or file it away for good, (2) make the hard stuff a 'task' or 'todo' inside of your mail program, (3) delegate stuff you shouldn't be doing, and (4) delete the rest. Be at less than five emails remaining in your inbox by the end of the day. I do it every day and so can you.

Show that inbox who's boss before you miss something from your boss.

3) Walking Tall

I know some people that'll circle around a building for a good ten minutes before they pick a parking spot. I have no idea why since they'd be in the building eight minutes earlier if they chose the open spot in the back. Plus, doesn't it seem like a nicer thing to do when there are folks that may be more tired, aged, or less mobile and need the closer spots more than you do? A few more steps in the parking lot gives you a few seconds to enjoy the beauty that is outside before chugging along inside.

Life always seems to be more enjoyable and beautiful when we slow down, stop to smell the roses, and begin to take in what's out there. Too often, we're focused on the most efficient, cost-effective, and easiest path. That may work for most things, but sometimes we need to slow down and soak life in. There's a lot out there to miss and it isn't always best to go flying through it.

Just Be Better: Park in the farthest parking spot from your office for two weeks. Alternate between two or three spaces in the general area so you don't get used to the same spot. Really enjoy the walk. Look at the landscaping, the clouds, and how pretty the weeds poking out of the cracks are.

Go a little slower and make life happen.

4) Boycott Email and Get More

I made the mistake of putting five of my personal email accounts on my phone and changed their checking frequency to every hour or so. I also turned on Facebook, Twitter, and other notifications. Can you imagine every time I looked at my phone I saw hundreds of little bugaboos winking at me? Oh my goodness. How am I supposed to work when I have all of these important things waiting for my immediate attention?

That's the big challenge. Is any of that stuff really necessary? Do you need to know what's going on in your outside-of-work life during your normal work hours? Don't you think if it's something very important, someone would actually pick up the phone and call you? Anyone who relies on any other form of communication besides the phone for an emergency is asking for trouble. Take back your attention and start working more effectively.

Just Be Better: Do not check your personal email, Facebook, or Twitter at all today. Don't even peek once. Turn your phone off if you have to. Do not make excuses when you eventually reply to the few people you missed. But I have a sneaking suspicion nothing Earth-shattering happened while you were gone.

Put the constant barrage of 'social' on hold. They can wait. You can wait.

5) Break Room Dancing

They had four different lunches in my high school days. Four! How they hee-haw was I supposed to sit with my three friends when they're split over four separate lunches? I thought that was a horrible idea and almost torture for nerdy kids like myself. It's hard enough to make friends when you're only interested in talking about Star Trek, Dungeons & Dragons, and programming. The last thing you want to do is take away those few hours with the friends you worked so hard to gain.

How things have changed. Or have they? How many people do you know at work? No, no, no. Not just how they work, what kind of details they catch and miss, or how well they can meet a deadline. I'm talking about really interacting with those who are around you for more than one-third of your weekdays. That's a good chunk of your life spent with people that are coworkers, but could also be called just acquaintances. How fulfilling are your work relationships, really?

Just Be Better: Bring your brown-bag lunch and eat in the break room today. Eat slowly. Be friendly. Bring extra goodies to share, offer a seat, and see what kind of awesome conversations you and your coworkers can strike up about non-work stuff. Hey, maybe talk about any new books you're reading.

Open up the doors to your world a little and see who comes in.

6) Relocation Vacation

For the past seven years, the space industry was a roller coaster ride. The space shuttle was officially retired, the space station has new contracts and no definite future, and there are tons of people caught in the middle. This sometimes leads to a constant barrage of requests, interruptions, and a sense of restlessness to meet constantly changing deadlines. It also results in a few empty cubes here and there. Can we combine these things and regain some control?

Change is hard. I don't know many people that enjoy constant change. Some view it as a threat to the status quo, that comfort we all know and have come to love. While others view change as yet another learning opportunity. Sometimes we have to take back control from drastic change in order to steer things in the right direction.

Just Be Better: Find one of those empty cubes from your latest wave of change. Sit at that new desk for four hours today and hammer out the project that needs the most attention. You might want to leave a sticky note at your main desk and let your boss know what you're doing, just in case. Be surprised with how much you get done in those four hours.

Use times of change to change the way you get more done.

7) Focus Like a Laser Beam

If you can coordinate the quiet time at home, teleworking can be an absolutely amazing experience. No one can drop by your cube for a surprise visit, no-one can dump a stack of papers on your desk, and there will be fewer calls to break up your focus. You have complete control over what you get done, how well it gets done, and how much time goes into getting it done.

Tweets, emails, texts, alarms, reminders, letters, and sticky notes barrage us from sun up to sun down. The human mind takes about six minutes to reset itself and refocus on the task at hand after an interruption. How many times are you interrupted throughout the day? Multiply that number by six and count up how much of your time is spent recovering from an interruption. Could you have gotten more work done without as many of those beeps and bloops?

Just Be Better: Okay so your boss won't let you telework. Fine. Here's the next step. Turn on the "out-of-office" notification setting in your email program today while you're at work. Put a note in the message asking people to call you if it's super important, otherwise you'll get back with them tomorrow.

Telework from work and get more done on your own terms.

Be A Better Person:

IN RELATIONSHIPS

Family is that inner circle that holds our deepest desires, fears, and memories. Everyone has a family of some sort and they all change so much throughout the years. Most families span four or five living generations of amazing experiences. How often do we look back at these folks with appreciation and thanks? They helped us grow from crawling on the floor to becoming the awesome people we are now. Let's see if we can give back a little more than we're used to.

8) Dining, No Whining

Family dinners were always great. Sure, you had a few snafus from time to time, but overall they were a wonderful time to catch up on old memories and see how things were going. But what about that last time you went out with only your dad or mom alone? Or what about your brother or sister? If it's been a while, you might not remember how intimate and awesome these experiences can be.

There's a huge break in the family dynamic when the kids leave the house for college, work, marriage, or the next big thing. Those bonds and comfort zones are immediately changed to something much less immediate. Something much less tangible and personal. Something distant, less frequent, and not as, well, family oriented. This is the logical next step in growing up, but how many of us take an extra step to refresh the bonds that got us where we are?

Just Be Better: Pick up the phone and ask a close family member out to dinner. Think of a couple of things to talk about ahead of time and plan to enjoy the heck out of it. Use this as a time to explore, grow, and see what their next step is. This is all about them. Oh yeah, and make sure you pay for the meal.

The bonds that bind us are the ones that made us. Respect the love.

9) Aunt You Gonna' Call Someone?

Have you ever got a call out of the blue by someone you haven't spoken to in a long time? You pick up your phone, see that caller ID, and wonder what's going on. I don't know about you, but my first reaction is usually hesitation. Not that I wouldn't want to talk to an old friend or family member, but it makes you wonder. I mean, why would anyone call out of the blue after being pretty much a stranger for such a long time?

We've all picked up some bad habits through our journey from being wild and crazy kids to being thriving adults. And along that crazy path, we've been busy growing, doing, moving, and shaking. But have we made enough time to maintain all of the close relationships we want to maintain? Sure, we have Facebook now and some of this dynamic is changing, but that's nothing compared to a good old, friendly, "no, I don't need anything I just want to talk" phone call.

Just Be Better: You might want to practice a few questions or topics ahead of time, but it certainly is not the main goal here. Call up the family member least likely to expect your call. Talk for at least five minutes about anything they want to. Be intimately interested in whatever they're up to at the moment. Keep it short, sweet, and totally friendly.

Try some close to home random acts of kindness.

10) No Chore in Keeping Secrets

Do you know what I'm not a big fan of? Vacuuming. It's far too much like mowing the lawn, except you don't get the great smells, outdoor adventure, and the thrill of a big spinning blade. Sure, the house is air conditioned and the vacuum is a lot easier to push around, but it just doesn't tickle my fancy as much. That's why my wife and I decided I do the yard and she does the floors. But that's also exactly the reason I sometimes do both.

We all have commitments we don't particularly enjoy. They're things we know we need to get done to keep our lives running smoothly, but they're the last things on our minds as far as motivation goes. How would you feel if you had a rough day with the kids, traffic, grocery shopping, cooking, laundry, and are starting to make your way to vacuum when you realize it's already done? Nothing to make a big deal about, of course, but what a nice little gesture. A nice little love gift.

Just Be Better: Pick a chore that you know another family member absolutely hates. Wait for them to go out and do something that will let you do your thing secretly. Now do that chore they hate and do it awesomely. Don't tell anyone and don't expect anything in return. Let it be a secret. Forget all about it.

Be a loving, chore-doing, secret admirer.

11) Honey, Do It Because You Love Me

Ever worked with those people that take extra effort to make sure you know how hard they worked to help you? Or how about the coworker that always has an excuse, comment, or ugly look whenever you try to ask them to help you out with something? Maybe there's a communication thing going on there, but talk about a horrible way to work through the day, right?

When's the last time you saw a successful doctor, nurse, or dentist with a super-crabby attitude? What's their secret to always being pleasant? How can they put up with the hundreds of different personalities and junk that gets thrown at them every day and still keep a healthy dose of cheer? They've latched on to something higher. They've found the real reason they do what they do and use it to propel them through all of the little junk that would grind anyone else to a halt. Something to be had there, my friend.

Just Be Better: Do whatever your spouse or significant other asks without any ugly faces, hesitation, or funky words. Do it because you love. Don't tell them you're doing it because of this exercise. Just do it out of the kindness of your heart and your realization that there's much more to life than wasting time being grumpy. It doesn't stick right away, but with practice it'll become a habit.

Honey always gets more attention than vinegar. Rub some honey on it.

12) Email: The Next Generation

I remember passing paper notes in school. We'd always get caught and then get embarrassed in front of the class but it was fun. Then I experimented with writing to a pen pal in Indonesia. That was a really cool experience. To have direct communication, to experience such a personal format, and choosing to cherish every letter was an awesome experience. Think about it. Those letters took hours to write, stuff, lick, stamp, and deliver. Each one was a piece of art, history, and your life.

So much of that is lost now with tweets, texts, and Facebook. Almost all communication hits the relationship pan with a flash and is gone forever. When's the last time you stared at a text message over and over again, day upon day, week after week? The folks that are hurting the most are the younger generations. I recently read that they hate email because it's too slow and takes too long. Really? It's time to start building up relationships and bring all ages together again.

Just Be Better: Send an email to one of your younger family members. Ask about their interests, what they like, what they plan to do in the next couple of months, and anything else you think your younger-self would've wanted to know at that age. Try to get at least 140 characters out of them, if you can.

Bridge the age gap and keep the communication appreciation going.

13) Flower Power

Okay, I'll admit it. I don't buy flowers for my wife as often as I used to. I'm definitely not proud of that fact, but I acknowledge I'll always have room to grow in showing my love for my wife. I make it a point to get lovely flowers on big days like St. Valentine's Day, our anniversary, and her birthday. But is that all? Isn't she worth a few random romantic reminders every once in a while? She did promise to put up with me for the rest of my life, after all.

We get comfortable. Extreme comfort in our jobs, friendships, relationships, and future. We often get to a point where we're content with what's going on. And instead of seeking to bring whatever it is to the next level, we try to keep the boat from rocking too much. Smooth sailing and avoiding those uncharted waters. It's all about the fear of the unknown, the fear of failure, and yes, even the fear of success. We know, deep down, when we put in the extra effort to grow our lives, that we'll eventually multiply everything.

Just Be Better: Buy one beautiful, love-capturing flower for the person you cherish the most. Don't expect anything in return. Not a thanks, not a hug, not a kiss. Nothing. Give and express your love from the innermost corner of your heart.

Build your relationships one flower at a time.

14) Inquiring Minds Want to Know

Remember that nerdy looking dude in your sixth grade class? You know, the one with the high-water pants, the out-of-style LA Gear pumps, and a cracked tooth? He never talked to anyone and he never seemed to have an awesome time outside of the schoolwork. That was me, by the way.

Often, we don't realize how much of an impact we can have in the lives of others if we choose to open ourselves up a bit. It's entirely possible to be completely alone in a room full of people. It's especially possible when you live alone and don't see your family for months or years on end.

Just Be Better: Hop in the car and plan a quick visit to an in-law or lesser-noticed family member for an hour. Work it into your next vacation if they live a little farther off. Talk about their life. Let them enjoy your listening ears and attention.

Give them time to share and give yourself time to grow.

15) No One Expects the Familial Inquisition!

We already covered the young folks in your family and how far they've come in the information revolution. But what about your oldest generations and where they're at? Do they tweet, text, or message in any other format than a phone call or a hand-written letter?

There's another big downfall to the progression of flash-communications. We leave those who don't adopt the new technology in the dust. More and more of the older generations are hearing and seeing less from their extended families. They don't get on Facebook, they don't send emails, and they probably don't even drive very far anymore. Let's fix this.

Just Be Better: Write a letter to your grandma or grandpa covering the highlights of your last year. Be humble, be respectful, and remember your audience. Ask them for advice and see what kind of life-long lessons you can learn from those excellent sources of wisdom.

Reach out and write someone, soon.

16) Love the Parental Units

I never understood how much my mom and dad did for me until my wife and I had our first kid. Especially after that first six months or so. Woo-boy, what a ride! The diapers, the no sleeping, the crying, the patience, the teaching, the doctors. Oh, the humanity of it all.

We tend to take for granted things we don't fully understand. A big fact of life is we don't understand much of any topic unless we actually have some experience with the topic. But, we can begin to appreciate and trust in those who've lived. They may not show it, but they know more than you can imagine.

Just Be Better: It's best if you do it in person, of course, but pick up the phone if you have to. Tell your mom and dad you love them. Be a little dramatic about it while being super genuine. Really put yourself in their position for a while and be deeply grateful for all they've done.

See the world from your parents' eyes and give them a nice little thankful surprise.

*****

Be A Better Person:

THROUGH GOD

There's a purpose and reason to everything you do. A lot of times we stop at the surface level without digging down deep to the real reasons. But if you ask the question "why?" enough times in a row, you will eventually reach the real reasons you do things. And you might find your real reason revolves around faith. Let's explore.

17) Be Strong, Be a Role Model

You know those really energetic and friendly waiters at your favorite restaurant? They always seem to have a great time and not worry about what others are thinking. Well, okay, they probably have good service and tips in mind, but not much stops their personality from shining through. They have the gumption to get stuff done in their own flavor. They choose to act. How do you choose to act in your own job?

Too often we shy away from sharing our real personality and feelings as a wall to protect our most sensitive insides. Not many folks can take an attack on their core values without feeling offended. But what if you could stay strong no matter what? What if you could be that shining role model that did the right thing in tough times? What would the right kind of people say?

Just Be Better: We have it easy in America. We can show our faith openly without anyone attacking us. Other countries don't have it so easy. The problem is we don't do it enough. Publicly give thanks for your meals. It will feel weird at first, but it's worth it. The trick is to pay attention to who you're really talking to.

Don't try to change the world; set the example.

18) Reflecting Porch

Ding! Mommy! Beep! Daddy! Tweet! Excuse me! Dong! HONK! Got a minute? Whoop! You have new email!

Any of these sound familiar? We have very busy lives and are constantly interrupted no matter where we go. We've turned from a society of hand-written letters to a global community of always on, always reachable techno-gurus. What happened to our time?

Slow down a bit. Do you ever get the feeling you're running at 800 mph or maybe you don't get enough of the important things done? Constant interruptions and a lack of real reflection time can grind you to a halt. Doing, working, and going at high speeds in everything you do will eventually lead to a crash. You've got to turn inside and shut out the outside every once in a while to recharge your spiritual batteries.

Just Be Better: Go out in the backyard or porch and quietly reflect on life for ten minutes. Don't try to make this time 'useful' by multitasking or by doing anything else. Leave your phone inside.

Slow down and gain time to catch up.

19) If You Don't Have Anything Nice to Say

I once heard someone say they'd rather be trapped on an island with a devout Buddhist than a lack-luster Christian. I agree. Think about it. Have you ever met a person who was truly devoted to their faith? They're sometimes hard to spot. They don't pressure you, they don't try to change your life, and they only discuss their faith with an open minded audience. Now the lack-luster folks, they want to push their beliefs on you while dismissing yours. Not cool.

What do you think happens when you try to talk about the most important thing someone believes in? Do you think you have a perfect grasp of what they believe or what they do? If they've been studying and believing their faith for a lifetime, where does your "outside view" fit in? You can't run into someone's home and start rearranging the furniture without causing some waves. They'll call you when they want your help. Be ready to answer.

Just Be Better: It's time to put on your "completely understanding" hat. Don't talk down, bad, or mean about any religion for three weeks. Go silent if you have to. I'm not asking you to change your beliefs. I'm asking to you appreciate strong values in everyone.

Faith comes from within and shows without. Be an admirer.

20) Random Inspiration

I have a good reason every time I say no to my son's request for candy. Don't get me wrong, treats are great and have their place, but they should be a rare and special thing. He may not understand why I say no on any particular instance, but he has come to accept that I'm true to my word and will make good decisions. But, that doesn't mean I won't respond to a random request at just the right time.

Faith is not a slot machine. No matter what you read out there, you can't look to the sky, ask for a million dollars, and expect the bills to start raining down. But, you can ask, open yourself up for the answer God has for you, and choose to make the answer work in your life. You don't know what's best for you, but He does.

Just Be Better: Grab your nearest Bible, open it up to a random spot, point your finger to any old place on the page, and read at least one verse. Slowly. Really digest the words. Roll them around in your head and heart. Close your eyes and see what pictures you see. How could this apply to your life?

Open your heart and learn to see the world from His point of view.

21) Pray From the Heart

Have you ever caught yourself saying something funky or mean about someone? I'm talking about random folks, too. That guy who just cut you off in traffic? Your boss when he asks you to stay late? You get my drift. If you started to count the number of times these things happened, you might be surprised what you find out.

When has any negative thought ever made your life better, besides allowing you to let off a little steam? Well, what if you could change the way you let off steam? What if you could focus your steam into an engine for doing something positive? What if you could turn your thoughts into a vehicle of prayer for that person instead?

Just Be Better: Say a short prayer for a person in need or a person you don't like. This is terribly hard at first, but it catches on real quick. Don't do the "well, BLEEESSS YOOUUU!!!" thing. Calm down for six seconds first and then pray genuinely for that person's wellbeing.

Taste the words that leave your mouth and bless the lives of others.

22) Quote Me Daily

It's hard to remember to take out the trash, clean the sink, or put the mail in the mailbox. These are things we know we need to pay attention to on a daily basis, but they tend to slip our immediate train of thought. Until we make them habits. The same goes for praying and paying attention to the gifts the good Lord has given you.

What's the second thing on your mind after you wake up? I already know what the first is so I won't ask. After my several bouts with cancer, I've gotten in the habit of being thankful for having another chance to see daylight. Thankful for being able to do another day's worth of good before the next day rolls around should I be so blessed. By keeping my mind continually reminded of what a gift a new day is, I start to focus on all the gifts given to me throughout the day.

Just Be Better: Keeping a small piece of God on your mind, daily, is the start of a good relationship that will always lead to more. Subscribe to a religious "quote of the day" email service. I'm partial to the **Minute Meditations and Saint of the Day folks**:

http://www.americancatholic.org/e-news/enewsletter-signup.aspx

Let the inspiration come to you and start your day out right.

23) Be Quick, Get Help

You know those people who always seem to know the right thing to say at exactly the right time? How do they do it? Do they just go home and practice responses day in and day out until they have every base covered? Or is there something else there that gives them the edge in being always present, always on top of things, and always ready to communicate with power?

The wheels of your brain machine get a little squeaky when they're thrown off track. Frustration, difficulty, and anger can throw us so far off balance that our usual systems don't work properly. Lashing out, saying the wrong thing, or just giving up are the last thing you want to do. But do you know you have other choices? There are other choices that actually help you grow.

Just Be Better: When you get frustrated, say a quick prayer for help. Make it something easy to remember and bring to mind at the blink of an eye. Something like, "God, please help me." Or maybe try, "Jesus, thank you and I love you" whenever you feel like it, too.

What you focus on focuses you. Focus on Infinite Love.

*****

Be A Better Person:

BY BEING HEALTHY

If you've ever tried to cut a tomato, you know a dull knife won't do the job. You've got to keep the tool in shape to get the job done properly. The same goes for your work and life. The food you eat, the exercise you get, and the physical rest you get are all part of your bigger energy picture. Start being a better person through living a healthier life.

24) Micro-No

I have to admit, running through a drive-through restaurant on those super-busy days is a real time-saver. But it's a huge hit to my health and builds my "I don't want to do anything" factor for the rest of the evening. You might say the convenience now makes the rest of my day inconvenient.

You might be surprised to find out the same goes for your home meals, too. Do you typically avoid bigger, fancier, or better meals because they can't be done quickly in the microwave? When's the last time you had to plan out a meal two or three hours in advance? It's a huge shift in healthy thinking and really gets you to appreciate the input, process, and output.

Just Be Better: Don't use your microwave at all for two full weeks. Not to boil water, not to heat up your oatmeal, not to reheat your coffee, not to destroy your CD's – nothing. Unplug it and move it to the garage. Seriously. Avoid the temptation and figure out other ways to make life work.

Start caring more about what goes into your meals and start getting more out of them.

25) A Spoon Full of Sugar, Gone

Those trips to the Chinese buffet are both wonderful and evil at the same time. One plate full of the best fried stuff, followed by the sweet and tasty meaty stuff, then a final round of the yummy dessert stuff. Oh and don't forget the sushi, egg-drop soup, and a few sugary-biscuits for good measure. Bite after bite after bite...

Once you hit your taste buds with something super fancy, you should consider the rest of the meal or snack downhill from there on out. That's how eating, and sometimes your whole day, can go. By not putting some extra care into your eating habits, you might leave that door open for unhealthy eating.

Just Be Better: Make your "food I don't need" bucket a little less full. Eat one less unhealthy item today. Ditch that piece of candy, ice cream, spoonful of mayo, and (as much as it hurts me to say it) those delicious slices of bacon.

Put a little less fuel on the junk-yard fire and boost your healthy eating journey.

26) An (Extra) Apple a Day

My wife and I took our son to Disney Land for his fourth birthday. He's a leap-year baby and it seemed like the right thing to do. That's a twelve hour trip from our house. I had a choice for fueling my driving energy. Do I start with candy, junk food, and sodas or trail mix, nuts, and juice? I've tried the junk food method before and can make it about an hour before I start falling asleep. I chose the good food method this time and I was fine the entire trip.

Beginning your trip to eating healthy is much easier when you start it off with the right kind of food. An old computer programming saying goes something like, "Garbage in, garbage out." The same goes for healthy eating and healthy starting. Put good stuff in and get good stuff out.

Just Be Better: Actively choose to eat one additional healthy item each day this week. Make it a banana, grapefruit, washed raw spinach, or even a handful of toasted almonds.

Start doing something different and build the good snack habit.

27) 10 Minute Abs-olutely Doable

Ever tried to run a few laps around the neighborhood park or running track? I know I've attempted it a few times myself. And there's one thing that kept me from doing it regularly. Time. I would spend ten minutes getting ready, thirty-five minutes exercising, and ten minutes cooling off and coming home. I couldn't cut a big enough piece of my day to do it regularly.

Then one day I bought a Gazelle. No, not the animal –
though chasing one would probably work up a big sweat.
It's an affordable elliptical machine I can use in my
home. In other words, I spend two minutes stretching,
twenty-five minutes exercising, and two minutes to cool
off. Bingo! Efficient exercise achieved.

Just Be Better: Take the at-home, anytime-is-good,
super-easy-to-do approach to exercise to get that habit
going. Exercise for at least ten minutes today. Stuck for
ideas? There are tons of ten-minute exercise videos on
YouTube. Try **this one**, **this one**, or **this one** to get
going.

http://www.youtube.com/watch?v=r_J8btnIEKQ
http://www.youtube.com/watch?v=ZlX_Gy4HP2E
http://www.youtube.com/watch?v=PWEdJRRndkQ

Get your body moving and give away the "no-time"
excuse.

28) Early to Bed

I've come up with so many different ways to justify
hitting the snooze button, it's sad to think about. I know
full well the extra nine minutes will do me no good and
will only shift my morning routine out of balance by the
same amount of time. But the desire to do it still comes
up. Silly.

You know sleep is vital to your energy and recovery. But
do you know just how important it is to start the next
day off right? If you tint your day with sluggish,
reluctant, and permissive habits, how do you think the
rest of the day will go?

Just Be Better: Get to bed eighteen minutes early today. Honestly consider getting double your snooze-time up front instead of in the morning when you don't have the extra time. It might be a little tougher for the first week. Keep at it and sleep will come with ease soon.

Take care first and start out right later.

29) Yes, Aspirin Does Expire

What joy is there in finding an old soda in the pantry? And I mean a really old one. You know it's going to be flat, funky, and just all kinds of bad. But you go for it anyway. Totally not worth it, especially considering you know better. But it's something you're in the habit of doing. Using what we've paid for, solely because you've bought it and it's there.

Consider this. If you bought an eighteen-pack of cookies for $2.99 and they're 470 calories each, would it be worth it, health-wise, to eat them just because they're there? How much time, money, and energy does it take to work off that $2.99? Would it be worth it to drink seven year old cough syrup knowing it's ineffective after the expiration date?

Just Be Better: Go through your medicine cabinet, bathroom, fridge, pantry, and drawers. Yank all of your expired pills, food, sauces, onion ice cream, and other junk. Dispose of them quickly and properly.

Start thinking about the cost of your future health before hanging on to money spent in the past.

30) Unblock the Sun

There's this recent habit of folks using vitamin supplements to cover all of the bases. Yes, I take a multivitamin for those days I know I'm not going to eat optimally, but there are things I won't do. For instance, I won't take vitamin D.

Your body was made to produce vitamin D from the get-go. Vitamin D is a vital nutrient for your health from everything to boosting immunity to preventing bone-softening rickets. And the best part is all you need is fifteen to twenty minutes in full sun to make it yourself. Neat, huh?

Just Be Better: Spend fifteen minutes in the sun today. You don't need sunblock for this unless you plan to stay out longer. Take a break, take some deep breaths, and enjoy the outside for a nice little chunk of time. Your body will thank you.

Bring some sunshine into your life and keep your body happy.

31) Dinner's Tough; Take a Nap

There's nothing like a good cup of coffee to round out a nice meal. It goes right in, fills in those empty spots in your stomach where the food couldn't reach, and makes you all nice and cozy-warm. It's a nice boost to energy, too. And it only takes about twenty minutes for the boost to kick in.

I admit eating can be a lot of work. All that chewing, talking, and moving about. Your body is doing so much and really needs to focus on turning that food into something you can use. In fact, it's so much work, something about a good meal just screams "nap-time!" So which is it? Nap or coffee?

Just Be Better: Do both. Grab a quick cup of coffee right after your dinner and then plunk down for a twenty minute nap. Set the alarm just in case. Play some **soothing music** or **guided relaxation audio**, if needed. Enjoy that break. You get a nap and will wake up right when the coffee is kicking in.

http://www.sky.fm/play/nature
http://www.youtube.com/watch?v=mrR2uaTNjTE

Stop fighting the after-meal dip and start using it for a double boost of energy.

32) Stop the Noise

Do you know what happens when you give a young kid a soda, a handful of chocolates, and let them loose? Small tornados of terror. And don't think adults get off the hook that easy either. Fill us with extra time on our electronic toys, time-wasting websites, and big-screen TV's and we're wired for hours.

When is there time to wind down in your life? You hit the ground running in the morning, fill the day with as many things as you can get done, and cool-off at the end of the day with doo-dads that occupy valuable mind-refreshing-time. You've got to rest before you can hit the hay.

Just Be Better: Turn your computer, phone, TV, and whatever else off two hours before going to bed today. Give your brain time to process the day, review your experiences, and learn from everything that happened.

Soak in the day's lessons before going to bed and sleep well.

33) Time Well Spent

Ever wonder where the time goes? Just as soon as you get home, there are 817 things waiting for you to do, right? By the time you've actually made a nice dent in the chores, you're staring at 10:00 PM without much time left before having to go to bed. Talk about a major drainer!

Chances are you don't have much control over what fills your day. You've got to work, take care of your family, and pay the bills. However, you do have control over what you do in your free time. Yes, I know certain things relax you over others. And what if I told you that other things could be just as relaxing and healthier at the same time?

Just Be Better: Start using your free time for more meaningful things. Cut back on your favorite game, website, or television show by at least thirty minutes today. Do something fun and rewarding in its place, but pick something to grow your skills or knowledge. Start the hobby you always wanted to, but only in thirty minute chunks.

Small chunks of time, repeated often enough, equal a lifetime of growth.

*****

Be A Better Person:

BY LEARNING

What's the difference between a young adult and a seasoned senior besides age? Their wisdom and experience. These are two things you can't think up and have. You have to live, experiment, and learn throughout your whole life in order to reach new levels of knowledge and expertise. The best time to start learning useful new things is yesterday. The second best time is today.

34) What's a Library?

I can't figure out why people aren't as excited about learning new things as me. I like to believe they're excited, but maybe not with the way things are taught now-a-days. Or is it that we're just moving so fast we don't think we have time to learn something new? Maybe it's the lack of a personal "educational fund" to buy books, training, or tickets to seminars? Or maybe it's a lack of awareness of all the awesome stuff that's out there?

Let's face it. If you're not motivated and looking for a new skill to learn and build, you'll never lift a finger in that direction. It boils down to motivation. If we're not excited about overcoming hurdles in our way, then why would we even bother learning how to do it? Sure, deep down we all know that there's more to be had, but what's wrong with what we have right now? Nothing. Nothing at all. Except everything. Everything you're missing.

Just Be Better: Go to your local library's website. Pick a random book. Check it out. Read for at least fifteen minutes. Or better yet, most libraries now have audiobooks available for free. You can be 'reading' while you drive to work, exercise, or mow the lawn. There's no reason you shouldn't be learning something. I learned a ton from almost 100 audiobooks in 2011. All free, thanks to my local library.

The growth is there for the taking. Be the reason.

35) Archive Party

I have this box of goodies I've kept since high school. It's got little notes, ticket stubs, silly little knick-knacks, printed (!) pictures, and other assorted things from my earlier days. I don't do it often, but it sure is nice to rummage through this box every once in a while. Especially the stuff that captures my thoughts and dreams from those days. Things have changed so much.

Being held back by your past is not a useful skill. However, reflecting on how you thought and planned for the future can be very useful. If you seek to learn from your past so that you can change your future, then you're on the right track. How have you changed since high school? How about since five years ago? Three years ago? One year?

Just Be Better: Review your personal notes, papers, and filed away goodies from the last year for at least twenty minutes today. Find the good stuff you have tucked away in the box in the attic or closet. Don't have anything? Try your super-old emails in the "Sent" folder in your email program. Start a new notebook or journal now so you'll have something to use for next year.

Look back and learn so you can go forward and earn.

36) Google Flogged My Noggin

A little over a decade ago, I remember having to do some research in my school's library. Yup, look up the books on the computer indexing system, find the book, and then skim through it until I found what I needed. Hardly fast, but it worked just fine. It's so much easier today. It's too easy, in fact.

It's so easy now I think people don't even bother looking stuff up anymore. Okay, okay - I get it. Not everyone likes to go to the library or read books. Fair enough. It's a fast world and we're all about having our answers right now. It's a good thing we have such a vast global resource available to us in the internet. But we need to use it more effectively to grow. There's so much out there, it's time to focus.

Just Be Better: Spend fifteen minutes "Google researching" a topic you're interested in. Just put that topic in the search bar with the words "how do I..." or "10 tips about..." and see what you come up with. Write down at least three interesting facts on an index card.

Make it a point to keep looking. Find something you like, plant the seed, and make it grow.

37) Define Simplicity

I'll admit I have no problem following along in a good technical book about learning, how the mind works, or advanced psychology. But sometimes, it's too much and I have to take a break. I give a lot of credit to those who can deal with five-dollar words day in and day out. It's very taxing.

But here's the kicker. After writing hundreds of thousands of words for many websites, several books, and countless emails, I can tell you one fact most people won't admit. Being simple is hard. Being simple is real hard. It's something that only comes with experience. Now's a good time to start.

Just Be Better: Go spend some time at **WordNet**. Look up three words you've had trouble with in the past. Digest the simplicity of the definitions you get there. Give yourself permission to use these words again.

http://wordnet.princeton.edu/

Start making your life simpler and start making more sense.

38) Grow Yourself Locally

Books, websites, email newsletters, videos, tweets, and more. There's no shortage of self-help or self-improvement gurus out there. And why not? It's such a great field with infinite room for growth. People need help and we always have another level to achieve, no matter how far we've gone.

But sometimes the plain text, lifeless video, or boring emails just don't cut it. There's just something about learning from people who actually practice what they teach in the real world that makes all the difference. Granted, public speaking isn't for everyone, but the ones that get it, get it good.

Just Be Better: Search for a local personal development or skills building seminar in your area. Plan to go. And then go. Take notes. Learn how to get to the next level in your life. Review your notes the following week. And then again a month later.

Real people are the secret sauce in growing.

39) Learning is Fun?

Now not all learning videos are boring. It takes a good team of writers, planners, technical folks, and enthusiastic actors to get a good thing going. There's a lot of decent stuff out there. However, you can only get so much "decent stuff" before you're tired of looking for learning all together.

So much of today's education isn't done with the human brain in mind. Most schools and teachers take the old-school methods that were designed to treat one kid the same as all others. But this doesn't work. Multiple intelligences, differing personalities, unique learning styles, and varying growth phases all come into play. But they all have something in common. Well researched, well prepared, and well executed material hits home every time.

Just Be Better: Go to the **VSauce YouTube channel**. Pick any video. Seriously, it doesn't matter which one you pick, they're all fantastic. Be amazed while you learn brand new subjects in less than seven minutes.

http://www.youtube.com/user/Vsauce

Hit education where it hurts and start having fun learning.

40) A Learning Frame of Mind

Ever tried to pick up a textbook, flip to a random page, and just start reading? I think I have. The thing is, I don't remember what I read when I do it that way. I wonder how many folks do this kind of studying for their school work or professional duties. All I know is it doesn't work, and boy do I feel like I wasted my time when it happens.

Learning is like exercising, you've got to warm up before you can take off. The brain is an absolutely wonderful machine, but it needs to be eased into new material. Some of this easing and preparing can be done with relaxation and mental preparation techniques. You're going to use your mind to learn, but you've got to use your mind to prepare, first.

Just Be Better: Practice getting into a learning frame of mind. It only takes about six minutes. Go check out my video on getting into **the learning state**. Practice it a few times and then get good at doing it on your own before big study sessions. Notice changes in your learning as you go forward.

http://www.youtube.com/watch?v=jzJNXcGDzRg

To learn, you must learn how to prepare to learn.

41) Fire in the Belly

How many times did you put off doing homework as a kid because your friends wanted you to come out and play? Or maybe you had a new video game you couldn't wait to put the smack down on. Either way, the last thing you were interested in was doing work. Especially learning.

And there's the real problem with that scenario. Learning isn't work, unless you make it work. If you're a die-hard fan of mowing the lawn, then dog gone it you're going to love mowing the lawn. Deep down, when you love to learn, you have a burning need to learn. A need that needs to be quenched. The same goes for everything you do or want to do. Find the motivation to turn work into play.

Just Be Better: Go figure out what motivates you to get stuff done. I've got a **free Self-Motivation Quiz** on my site that'll help. Now start using that type of motivation to get stuff done.

http://richardstep.com/self-motivation-quiz-test/

Light that fire and take off. It's time to want to learn and grow.

Be A Better Person:

THROUGH SUCCESS

"Success" is one of those wishy-washy words that most people think only means money, and lots of it. Maybe that's a good enough definition; maybe not. It could also mean being better with what you have, having a greater reach in your community, and how many people you've empowered across the globe. That seems hard to grasp for most folks, so let's go for something more practical and attainable. Let's hit up some small successes first.

42) Brown Bag Millionaire

Never mind how many pounds it made me gain, but I used to eat out for lunch every single weekday. No, nothing like a salad or a sandwich, either. We're talking the full deal Mexican meal, twelve ounce pork chop, Chinese buffet, and whatever else crazy idea came across my coworkers' minds. Can you imagine what fifteen-dollars per day looks like at the end of the year? That's getting real close to $4,000. Four grand, can you believe that? Three times the raises I earned in corporate America went straight to my gut.

We get so used to pumping out money for things we're convinced we need. I mean it's food, right? We have to eat, right? Do we have to have a party each time? Moderation is a common theme when it comes to eating habits. There's a reason we don't eat German chocolate cake for dinner every day, as good as it sounds.

Just Be Better: Go about as caveman-esque as you can and bring a brown-bag lunch to work for a week. I'm talking about grabbing a loaf of wheat bread, jar of organic peanut butter, some raisins, and some cheapo crackers. Count up how much money you didn't spend that week.

As a guide, I ate mostly healthy and hearty $1.23 lunches for three years while bootstrapping my personal business ventures. That comes to about $310 in lunches for one year, which is less than ten-percent of the $4k lunch-meal plan. I ate lunch for one year from what I used to pay in the $4k-lunch-meal plan taxes alone.

Regain control of your intake, and snag a few thousand for your wallet.

43) Cut It Out

My wife and I decided to go on a twenty-five-dollars-per-month allowance right after we got married. You want to talk about tough? What the hee-haw could I buy for twenty-five dollars? It took me four months to save up for some photo editing software. By then it was almost time for the new version to come out. But you know what happened? I started learning how to plan, spend, and best of all, not spend.

There's a phenomenon called "lifestyle creep" that hits people hard whenever they get a bump up in the money they earn. I've read articles of people that earn millions per year but are broke because of their habits. Your tastes and habits can make you a millionaire pauper if you don't have a good set of rules in place.

Just Be Better: Make a list of things you buy, but don't need. This is the random DVD or CD at your local electronics store, the sale items at the clothing store, and the extra bag of fancy candies at the checkout lane. Cut one of the needless things, or wants, out for at least one month. Be fair to yourself and pick something you usually buy often. Now stop it cold turkey.

Your bank account is a bucket; plug the leaks.

44) Auto-Barista

I never used to drink coffee and I didn't understand what the big deal was. Until I started my last few years in college and pulled multiple all-nighters. Wow. What a jolt to my immediate energy levels and mental powers. Coffee was like a mysterious super-power juice waiting to propel me to the next level. I was sold. Sold a bit too much, actually. That dog-gone Starbucks place took a fair share of my hard earned Ramen noodle dollars, I'm sorry to admit.

How often do we pick up something we think we need, when we could do the same at home for one-tenth the cost and almost the same amount of time? We get in the habit of convincing ourselves certain services save us time and convenience at the cost of a higher price. Well guess what, stop kidding yourself and start taking back your ability to manage time and money.

Just Be Better: Make your own coffee for three weeks. Don't have the goodies? It's sixteen bucks for a cheapo four-cup coffee machine, six dollars for twelve ounces of a decent coffee that will last three weeks, and ten dollars for a thermal container to keep it warm in. That's thirty-two dollars in three weeks for coffee you control compared to eighty-dollars for coffee you get served.

And the "at home" option only gets cheaper with time since you already have the machine and thermal container. Think you don't have time? Let it brew while you take a shower; problem solved.

Be your own barista. Tip well.

45) A Percentage of Riches

Remember when I talked about the little wants we pick up here and there? You know, the five-dollars here, the two-dollars there, and the occasional ten-dollars over there. You're punching holes in your bank bucket one unneeded thing at a time and you don't even know it. It's like sharing a bag of popcorn at the movies. You don't notice how much is left until there's nothing left. Watch out.

Humans aren't capable of quantifying large groups of things. When we see a big group of people, numbers don't pop into our minds anymore as we jump straight to a broad generalization of, "a lot of people." It isn't until the crowd is down to a manageable five or so people that we start thinking in numbers. The same goes for money and time. We think we have so much of it, until we don't.

Just Be Better: Let's flip this idea over and see how we can benefit from it. Put one percent of your next paycheck into a savings account. If the company you work for allows you to do it automatically, even better. You won't miss it. Repeat often.

The details hide a lot. Pay yourself first and save for the future.

46) Just One Step

I remember the days of thinking about writing a book. I knew I wanted to do it. I knew I wanted to leave my mark on the world and share with those patient enough to wade through it. But where the heck would I begin? I didn't know anything about writing a book. I was effectively paralyzed by being overwhelmed by my lack of knowledge.

This happens a lot more than people want to admit. Why don't we go for that training class on something we're passionate about? Why don't we volunteer for things that will move us forward? Why don't we take more chances and see what happens? Too often, we think too much and do too little. Now's the time to reverse that thinking.

Just Be Better: Write down your biggest goal on a blank sheet of paper. Write at least fifteen ways to achieve that goal. It's okay if some of them are silly or too hard to do. Just write. Next, write down the very next "fifteen minute" step you can take toward finishing the goal. The smallest little chunk of a step to move your forward. Now take that step today.

The hardest part of getting a train moving is getting it started.

47) Magic Money Rules

Wondering what to do with the thousands of dollars you've saved in lunches, coffee, and doodads you don't need? It's time to take it to the next level. The problem is, what's the next level? Do you shove the money in the bank, rack up the measly fraction of a percent in interest that doesn't beat the three percent inflation rise every year, and then wait? Wait for what?

One of the biggest problems about money saving, making, and expanding is awareness. Not enough people realize there's magic involved when it comes to maximizing their income. Success and growth are all about leverage - getting the most out of what we have. We have to find more ways to make everything we do mean so much more.

Just Be Better: Bust out your favorite search engine and look up the "magic of compound interest" and the "rule of 72." Give it a day or so to sink in. Now see how these two ideas can work for you if you would put your extra $4,000 into something more financially useful. Now, make financial plans accordingly. Call a professional if you have to. If you don't, the $300 service fee they charge will be lost in the money you don't earn from the interest you could have earned in one year.

Get more bang for your buck by learning the basics of earning.

48) Financial Brushing

I cherished those long days when my family and I played Monopoly™ for hours on end. They used to think I was crazy for buying up as much property as I could. I mean heck, I would have almost no money in my hands, just a bunch of property cards. Fast forward a few hours and it all started to make sense. Landing on hotels every roll of the dice starts to hurt your bank reserves when you're a guest and not an owner.

I normally blame it on society and the media, but most folks have a hard time delaying investment gratification for more than a year. A decade ago this average "investment holding period" was five years. Did you know the chance to lose money goes to almost zero percent after ten years in most stable, low-fee stock market index funds? Did you also know the average rate of return is anywhere from seven to eleven percent for those same funds, when properly distributed? Get that rate at your bank, I dare ya'.

Just Be Better: It's time to brush up on your finances and start making your money work for you. Are you a beginner and a bit confused by the process? Check out my notes on **Comfort Zone Investing**. Are you advanced, instead? Check out my notes on **The Intelligent Asset Allocator**. I highly recommend both of those books, too, if you have the time. They're worth the investment.

http://richardstep.com/downloads/tools/Notes--Comfort-Zone-Investing.pdf
http://richardstep.com/downloads/tools/Notes--The-Intelligent-Asset-Allocator.pdf

Stop being a guest and think of your dollars as employees. Now put them to work.

✳✳✳✳✳

Be A Better Person:

THROUGH CREATIVITY

Have you ever caught yourself saying something fun or relaxing is a waste of time? I know I have, especially when I'm deep in a big project and focused on getting stuff done. I have to remind myself a nice creativity recharge can do wonders for focus, ideas, and overall energy.

49) Army vs. Puffy White Things

There were two things I enjoyed playing with, and melting, when I was a child. Those funky little dark-green army figurines and big marshmallows. No, not the mini-marshmallows, those don't count. One represented the beginning of strategy and national security for me. The other stood for playful snacking and memorable eating. Both great fun, though one was tastier.

These are childhood memories embedded deep inside and you've probably never given them another thought since then. But you sure as hee-haw get flooded with fond memories when you see them again. Tapping into these good experiences can help you practice focusing on the good.

Just Be Better: What happens when we mix these two together? Draw a stick figure army attacking a big bag of marshmallows. Imagine what happens when an army figure gets engulfed by a marshmallow. Picture the mallow getting swarmed by a platoon. What happens? Want bonus points? Use the real things.

Draw from your childhood to bust boundaries and enjoy creative playing.

50) Home Sweet Crayons

Who doesn't remember converting all of their childhood memories into crayon and paper landscapes? The waxy smell, those weird color names, and the pain inside you when one accidently breaks while coloring. Crayons are such great tools with such great outcomes.

There's something to be had there. You didn't sit around trying to figure out what to draw. You just drew. You picked up the crayon, found a blank spot on the paper, and went at it. No doubts. No second thoughts. Just action. Simple tools didn't get in the way.

Just Be Better: Find a big sheet of paper. Find some crayons. Just start drawing anything. And since there's a big chance you'll spend too much time thinking about it (now that you're a "grown up"), here's an idea. Draw your childhood house. Close your eyes, get the picture inside, and scribble down a draft version of it. Bring it out and put it down. Don't forget the mailbox and shades on the sun!

Simple tools enable immediate action; get simple and get going.

51) Rough Purple Ideas

It's Saturday afternoon and your family is hungry. Do you go to the burger joint or the fried chicken place? Do you eat there or go home? Do you super-size or down size? What, oh what, should you do with these choices? How about something completely different?

You often go through the day doing things as you've always done them. These are mostly automatic patterns. You might not be aware there are other choices to add to your list. Other choices that could change your life or make it more enjoyable. Being able to find these choices is a skill you need to learn.

Just Be Better: Get a sheet of paper, fold it in half, write 'purple' on one side of the fold-line and 'rough' on the other side. List as many purple things on the 'purple' side and as many rough things on the 'rough' side as you can. Now combine one word from each side to get a new idea. Do this four more times. Look over your five new ideas and imagine something useful.

Look outside of the box of the familiar and see new possibilities.

52) More than Meets Your Eyes

There's nothing quite like laying down in the warm and crunchy green grass on a nice afternoon. A gentle breeze flowing over your skin. Your hands behind your head tilting your view to the perfect cloud gazing angle. Slowly watching the shapes in the sky transform into all kinds of interesting things. Relaxing. Refreshing. Awesome.

Sometimes the best way to recharge your creative juices is to let creativity happen to you. You can gain so much by going with the flow and taking advantage of the tons of creativity around you every day. Actively trying to notice these forces is an amazing idea.

Just Be Better: Go outside, lie down, and look up. Find at least three different objects in the clouds. Watch them slowly transform into dragons, stuffed animals, and pieces of pizza. Relax and let it flow.

Give yourself permission to enjoy life's creative flow.

53) Playing with Dough

Simple creativity tools help get your logical mind out of the way and let the creative mind come out and play. This is a good thing. Remember the simple tool you once loved for making a three dimensional play world? Smashing, rolling, and maybe even tasting was the name of the game when it came to play-dough.

Getting deep into the creative process is one step closer to getting your head out of the way and letting things flow. There's something fulfilling in diving into projects and play, getting your hands dirty and creating with reckless abandon.

Just Be Better: Do an internet search for "play-dough recipe." Get your ingredients together and make some. Play with it. Play with it for a long time. Relive your childhood and make those awesome things you used to make in the days when life wasn't as serious.

Get your hands dirty and shut off that nagging logical mind for a while.

54) Blossoming Solutions

Okay, I'll admit I used to be one of these people. You know the ones. They want to be and do so much but they keep defaulting to the same excuse: "I can't come up with any good ideas" or "I don't know what to do." This is understandable as most work environments don't help build the creative qualities in their folks.

But then I came to realize it's time for me to take my creative growth into my own hands. Everybody is unique and has a ton of varying preferences. I can understand why there's no real room for creativity growth in most office environments. It's a sad thing because opening up your mind to the infinite possibilities of life is so important for growth.

Just Be Better: The trick in growing your creative genius is to use tools to help focus your creative juices. Try the **Lotus Blossom brainstorming method** on a difficult problem you have around the house. Then do at least one of the ideas you come up with to fix it. Prepare to be amazed. Seriously.

http://richardstep.com/self-help/discover-64-ways-live-your-passion-less-than-15-minutes/

Creative growth worked for the first seven years of your life; do it again.

55) A Passionate Dish

So you're sold on brainstorming and growing your creativity now, right? That's good. Sometimes having only one tool to go to can slow you down in your creative growth. It's best to have choices when it comes to pulling ideas out of your infinite idea generator: your brain.

There are a ton of great brainstorming books out there and I will recommend anything by Michael Michalko until I'm blue in the face. He does a great job explaining and showing instead of just telling. Let me also point you to the **brainstorming section** on my website where I have quite a few methods and cheat-sheets available for free use.

http://richardstep.com/tools/brainstorming-methods/

Just Be Better: For now, let's try and make another tasty idea dish. Let's see if we can find your life passions through the **Fruit-Root-Tree brainstorming** exercise. It's quick and fun and will probably leave your mouth watering with possibilities. I've also got a **book** that goes into this line of thinking in more detail.

http://richardstep.com/creativity/passion-interests-new-fruit-root-tree-brainstorming-method/
http://amzn.com/B008T3V5H2

Dish out the ideas and start growing your life again.

56) Leaning Tower of Dough

Playing around and enjoying life are great things and will help you feel better, relax, and appreciate the comfort level you've gained. Want to take it up a notch for the fun and challenging factor? It's something we need to do to keep our minds and motivations fresh. All fun and no play, well, there's something to that.

Creative, useful, and practical play is a perfect combination of fun and output. What's a key difference between an entrepreneur and a cube-environment worker? An entrepreneur isn't working; she's having a dang good time solving problems for other people in exchange for time, resources, and freedom. She's doing something useful, fun, and beneficial for her personal empire. She's having fun and getting stuff done.

Just Be Better: Build your entrepreneurial spirit by having more fun getting useful stuff done. Let's start out small, though. Use the play-dough you made from before, along with some toothpicks, to make a tower. Try to touch the ceiling. That's the challenging goal for this fun exercise. You're not just playing; you're solving a problem and learning along the way.

Align yourself with a useful outcome and have a blast doing it.

Be A Better Person:

BY EXPLORING

We're best in all we do when we go into things without any judgments in mind and with a curious approach. What's the best way to get into this wonderful state of child-like awesomeness? Explore. Explore like you've never explored before. Open up the door of possibility and see what's on the other side.

57) Hunting for Four Leaf Clovers

Surely you've heard of the mysterious four leaf clover by now. A trophy-hunt told by many fun-loving adults to their lovingly fun children. These wonderful little plants are promised to give you years and years of good luck and great fortune. There's only one catch. They're extremely difficult to find.

Did that fact ever stop us from looking? Did we ever plop down on the ground and give up looking for a lifetime of good fortune and fun? Nope. We kept looking. We knew the odds were stacked against us but the hope was strong. The hope and work kept us going.

Just Be Better: Find a local park or low-traffic, green-space area. Get on your hands and knees and check out every square inch. Look for a plant you've never seen before. It doesn't have to be a four leaf clover, but you get bonus points if you find one.

Explore the world with new eyes, and make it your prize.

58) Guided Meditation

I thoroughly enjoy telling stories to my kiddos, whether the stories are from books or made up on the spot. There's something about the trance-like state of enjoyment they go into when story time happens. You know what I like even better than that? When someone else can get me that interested in something.

Meditation can be something as simple as a short prayer to God or as complex as experiencing your personality through meditating on the life-cycles of a butterfly. There's only one major problem; not many folks know how to do it. While the short prayer version is easier, the more complex version works great with some outside help.

Just Be Better: Search YouTube for a guided meditation exercise. There's a lot of decent stuff out there, but there are some awesome ones that will blow your mind with relaxing, purposeful exploration. Okay, okay, I'll pick – **try this one**.

http://www.youtube.com/watch?v=QT5w5rBUaxw

Get some help, explore yourself, and meditate on a better you.

59) Museums Have Lessons?

I remember enjoying those rare field trips when we would go to local museums. Sure, it was supposed to be school related in some way, but I didn't care. I got to get out of the classroom and hang out with my friends. That was the real point, right?

Every piece of art, decoration, arrangement, and letter in a museum has a purpose or meaning. The really old stuff is especially interesting. Can you imagine the people that carved that mask from 800 BC? What were they thinking while they whittled away at the log? Who was it for? How long did it take? Did the artist stick her tongue out in concentration during the carving?

Just Be Better: Hop over to the local museum or zoo. Go to every exhibit. Read the plaques. Walk away with at least five new facts or insights. Really dive into the whole story and see what you can find or make up.

Find the story in everything and be constantly amazed.

60) Wandering Aimlessly

Oh the feeling you get when you're lost. Add on the "late, tired, and hungry" feelings to it and you have a wonderful combination, right? Frustration is the main thing on your mind and you know no one is having any fun. Do you know anyone that's ever tried to get lost on purpose? It doesn't work that way for some reason.

What if we took the "bad stigma" out of the equation and focused on just the "lost" part? Would we really be lost or is "lost" just a word we use when we're exploring *and* frustrated? It's too bad. Exploring is only a quick change-of-mind choice away from lost. Maybe it's time to change the definition.

Just Be Better: Get in the car, point yourself in a direction, and drive. Put a sticky note over the clock, turn off your phone, turn off the GPS, and have no destination in mind. Go until you see something so interesting you feel compelled to stop. You can turn on GPS to get back home, if you must.

Go out of your comfort zone and zone out.

61) Pronounce This

I've come across a few lovely dishes I wouldn't have eaten if their names were in English. The funny thing is, they were absolutely delicious. Sure, I didn't know how to cook them but a friend or internet search was always a phone call or click away.

You might remember a story about some green eggs that came with some similarly colored ham, right? Why is it we've come to forget the point of the story? You've got to give new things a try before you shut them out of your life.

Just Be Better: Go to an ethnic grocery store. Buy at least three things you can't pronounce. Look up some interesting recipes online and use those things you bought to do a little experimenting.

Possibilities are a willing mind away; so will it already.

62) Eat It, I Dare You

Are you the kind of person that goes to seven different types of restaurants and orders the same Cobb salad, fish and chips, fajitas, or chicken-fried steak? It seems like no matter where you go restaurants cater their menus to folks looking for the safe and easy choice.

Comfort. Yes, I know it is a lovely and wonderful word. Unfortunately, it usually comes along with complacency and lukewarm-ness. We find a route we like and we tend to stick with it. It may have worked for us once before, but that doesn't mean it's the best route of all time.

Just Be Better: Go to a new restaurant and order something unfamiliar. Want to really go out on a limb? Ask the waiter to pick their favorite dish or maybe the house special. Do not order something you're familiar with.

Just try it, you might like it.

63) Howdy Neighbor

Think back to the last time you went on vacation or stopped in a small town on a road trip. How did you feel when you walked around the restaurants, grocery stores, or malls? Out of place? Curious? Adventurous? Special? Like you could do whatever you want and it wouldn't matter?

You might be amazed at how much your actions are determined by the people around you. You get familiar with people, you know they expect you to act a certain way, and you might choose to stick to that way to keep from stirring the pot. The question is, is this trend holding you back?

Just Be Better: Travel to a town near to you you've never been to. Walk around some of the stores and observe people. Chat up a few conversations and ask what's on their minds. Be interested, be interesting, and live life a little more.

Be better than you. Be a new you. Be the new you that you want to be.

*****

Be A Better Person:

THROUGH THINKING

I know no one reads directions anymore and product manuals are almost immediately thrown in the trash. But what happens when you get to the step when things don't seem to fit properly? It's time to get the instructions down right. You've got to fix the inside before anything will stick on the outside.

64) Mental Fist-Pumps

The further I get from the high school and college days, the more I realize I don't have the same emotional safety-net I once had. It's not worse, it's just not the same. I can talk to my wife and call up a buddy at the drop of a hat, but this doesn't seem to get it on some of the most difficult days.

Every entrepreneurial journey can be rough and lonely. You're busting your bum to hustle out as much useful content as you can on a limited amount of time. If you can't keep yourself going, no one else will. You've got to be your own fuel to keep your fire burning.

Just Be Better: Go ahead and give yourself permission to be cheesy. Cheer yourself on and congratulate yourself for little wins. Aim for at least five today. Mental fist-pumps are okay. You deserve it.

Every time you pat yourself on the back, you push yourself forward.

65) Unique Snowflakes

I didn't find this out until I was in my thirties, but my mom used to buy us clothes from Goodwill when we were in middle school. Do I think there is anything wrong with this? No, they have great stuff. Would my friends have cared? Maybe. Did I give two flying whoopity-doodads? Heck no.

The more we can get over caring about someone else's opinion of the way we look, the more we can start to focus on what matters in life. Being able to direct your own actions and behaviors based on your own judgments is key for guiding your life.

Just Be Better: Stop the "appearance judging" game, starting with yourself to build up your experience. Do not judge the appearance of anyone today. Catch yourself and just stop.

Some clothes are better than no clothes. Focus on what matters: the person inside.

66) Fixing the Unhappy

Ever gone on a hiking trip? What kind of stuff did you put in your backpack? It doesn't matter what was inside, but I can guess it was probably too much. In fact, if it was more than water and a knife for a day trip, it was too much. And guess what? The extra stuff weighed you down unnecessarily.

There are tons of things we don't need in our life's backpack. Constantly dragging it around when we know dang well it isn't doing us any good. We get used to the weight on our back and forget about it. Our strength returns once we drop the pack and move on.

Just Be Better: List the top three reasons you're not happy with something. It can be something big or small. I recommend aiming for something small and doable first. Think of three things you can do to fix each one of the unhappy things. Do one of those three things before next Sunday.

Lighten the load and enhance your happy – less weight, more hike.

67) Self Talk is Okay

Remember Jack Handey and his Deep Thoughts? Way overdone, way over-the-top, and easily dismissed as light humor. You know what real damage was done here? People immediately think any type of self-talk is useless as they think back to Jack's parodies, without realizing they were only parodies.

Auto-suggestion, also known as self-talk, has been given the **green light by psychology** since the Deep Thoughts era, when used properly. Yes, telling yourself you are a "unique snowflake" isn't helpful. But, it's powerfully enabling to remind yourself that you "have an infinite wealth of memories to look back on for ideas and solutions to your current problems." There's a huge difference and I suggest you use the latter one.

http://psychcentral.com/news/2010/09/22/self-talk-helps-self-control/18534.html

Just Be Better: Try out some positive, useful **self-talk exercises** today. See if you can stick with it for at least a week in a row. Then go for twenty-one days to make it a good habit.

http://www.youtube.com/watch?v=tU9islARUCA

You are your harshest critic and best supporter. Keep your messages uplifting.

68) Judge Not, Just Describe

Do you know someone who's "not attractive" or is that person just "someone *I* am not attracted to?" How about a coworker that's a "total grouch" or maybe "in a mood I don't fully understand?" Is anyone you know "short" or are they simply "four feet and ten inches tall?" Is that unruly kid over there too much of a "wild brat" or does he not "have the right emotional tools for dealing with this situation?"

Walls. What we build around ourselves are walls. Day in and day out we're all about putting up defenses, brick by brick. Why? To fend off the judgers. There's only one problem. The worst offender is inside. Your inner critic can turn something as simple as a number to describe your weight into something as depressing as a useless label.

Just Be Better: Turn something you think is negative about someone into a descriptive statement. Is someone you know really "fat" or do they just "weigh XXX pounds?" Do this two more times for yourself.

Just the facts, ma'am, just the facts. Your judgments are not welcome here.

69) Stop, Calibrate, and Listen

I know there are plenty of examples out there, but I'll stick with parenting because it's something I enjoy and am intimately familiar with. Ever sat and watched kids play with something they're not supposed to? Is your immediate reaction to stop, correct, and teach? Let them grow and experiment. It's your job to know when to step in. It's what child-rearing adults do to help their kiddos grow.

When does this constant calibration to what works in life finally stop? When can you finally rest in the lesson learning and useful thinking process? Never. Your parents won't do it for you anymore and now you have to be your own teacher, educator, calibrator, and correctional officer.

Just Be Better: Continue to pay attention to what you think. Catch yourself the next time you put yourself down or anyone else. Stop it. Replace it with something useful and positive, big or small. Replace the bad with good at least five times today. Keep doing it and get used to it.

The power to make a better you is in your hands and head.

70) The Most Interesting People in the World

You and I, we're the same, right? Both humans, both between four and eight feet tall, somewhere around 200 pounds plus or minus 100, and we both eat, drink, and sleep, right? But what about our insides? How we were raised, what beliefs we've come to hold close, how capable we think we are, what mistakes we've made, and the lessons we've learned?

If you want to begin to understand the concept of 'infinity,' try and think about every awesome thought you've ever had. And remember, what was awesome at two years old and is seen as silly now was still awesome from your frame of mind back then. Now, when you're done, think about how many awesome experiences your best friend has had over the years. This should take a while; take your time.

Just Be Better: Everyone has a story to tell, probably hundreds, and you don't know half of them. Pretend the people you talk with today are the most interesting people in the world.

Stay interested my friends; there's more to people than you think.

71) Cliché Olé

When's the last time you said "he is such a pain in the neck," "no sweat off my back," or "maybe when the cows come home?" Do you have any idea what those phrases mean or are they shortcuts for not having to think too much? Do you mean what you're saying?

You know words are very important. Too often, we use familiar phrases as a crutch so we don't have to spend too much time thinking of what we want to say. Do you know how many of those sayings and thoughts might be holding you back from trying something new?

Just Be Better: Think of your favorite or most often used cliché. Research where it came from and how it was originally used. Now decide whether or not you like what you've learned.

Do your own thinking and regain control.

*****

Be A Better Person:

BY HAVING FUN

Going through the grind is sometimes a necessary thing, but it can't be all that you do. If you want to add some spunk to your life, you'll need to keep your fun-bucket full. Turning everyday situations into opportunities to learn and grow is what this is about. Start being a better person by having more fun.

72) Drive-Thru Fancy

Some say the best way to get by is to fake it until you make it. Some say to make it until you break it. I say to go right in and take it. Okay well, not literally.

But think about this for a second. Why do we take pictures of animals at the zoo? Is it to jog our memories later? Is it to have evidence of our awesome adventure out? Is it to capture the beauty flowing in nature? Yes, yes, and yes.

Apply this memory capturing idea to your journey through enjoying life more, too. Do you get sad around rich people and their awesome stuff? Or do you bless them and appreciate the evidence they show that hard work really does pay off? Find inspiration in the success of others.

Just Be Better: Drive through the richest and fanciest part of town and just let it all soak in. Check out those awesome topiaries as you stroll by in your car. See how many Lamborghinis and Bentleys you can spot. Celebrate the beauty that comes with focused effort and energy. They're people made of the same stuff you are.

It's possible for anyone to succeed. Have fun learning from the successes of others.

73) Get Your (New) Game On

When I was growing up, there were only two board games we could play: Monopoly™ and Life™. We'd play the former when we had eight hours to burn and the latter when we wanted to play with little toys that wouldn't fit together properly.

Did you know there are hundreds of board games you've never heard of that absolutely blow these two board games out of the water? Neither did I, until I ran across a board game collector and this website he recommended: **http://boardgamegeek.com/**

Just Be Better: Make it your mission to find a new board game to bring into your home. Try **Lost Cities**™. It's super-quick, super-addictive, and simple. Be brave and try new ways to have fun at home.

Start playing games no one's ever heard of.

74) Get Your (Old) Game On

Ever sit around and daydream about your best playground experiences from childhood? How about the first time you won a game of Go Fish! Did picking up the last jack before the ball hits the ground, as your friend looked over in disappointment, give you a sense of accomplishment? Those are some great memories right there.

On a similar note, when's the last time you actually played Monopoly™ or Life™? Or how about Mouse Trap™, Sorry™, Backgammon, Othello, Chess, Chinese Checkers, Risk™, or Guess Who? These are some of the staples of childhood gaming.

Just Be Better: Go out there, find the oldest board game you have, and gather enough people to play. Send out the invites, grab some snacks and drinks, and have the best dang "Board Game Throw Back Party" you ever had.

You played to live back then; now replay to relive again.

75) Make Bad Movies Good

Where you ever stuck in a situation you couldn't stand? Something like your car broke down, the front tire popped, a headlight went out, and it's raining? There's not much you can do in that situation other than throw your hands up and let the chips fall where they may. Or, you can choose to make it more useful than it seems to be.

It's the low and frustrating times when we can truly start growing. It isn't until we've been thrown into the fire and rolled around a bit that we finally see what matters in our lives. I don't want you to purposefully pop your tires to learn a lesson, but there are good opportunities you can safely create yourself.

Just Be Better: Go see a movie and I mean pick the worst one you can. Every movie you've ever seen been a total winner? Let's pick a total loser. How about grabbing "Superbabies: Baby Geniuses 2" (2004). Watch it with a completely open mind knowing, for a fact, that it will absolutely stink to high Heaven. Choose to make it fun while you watch. You might even try doing what the **Mystery Science Theater 3000 folks** did.

Safely experience the bad so you can grow your ability to find the good.

76) Playground Flashback

There's nothing like sitting at the top of a bright yellow slide, hanging on for dear life, as your knuckles go white in anticipation. The line behind you is piling up and you know you have to go, but you want one more minute to soak it all in. You push off and spiral down, wind rushing by your face, feeling like a true dare-devil. Do you miss the playground days?

The routine of daily operations can wear on you from time to time. Sure, bills and responsibilities are priority, but do they have to be the only things getting attention? Your mind and soul need an extra boost of play-time to recover. There's nothing like breaking the grind for a few hours to recharge your batteries.

Just Be Better: Go to a playground nearby and play your heart out. Afraid you'll be a little embarrassed? Bring a kid if you need an excuse. Surely you've got a relative that could use a babysitter for an hour or so. They'd love the offer. While you're at the playground, be sure to swing above the bar and avoid the lava.

Relive those peak playground experiences and put life into perspective.

77) Cheer Leading

Have you ever done something you thought was an awesome accomplishment, but there was no one around to share it with? Or maybe those who were around cared a little less than you did? Sometimes, your accomplishments can be drowned out by all of life's noise and by the competition for attention by others.

When you continue to neglect the good feelings that come with being recognized for doing great work, the effect begins to dull. When the effect dulls, the motivation can dwindle. You've got to keep motivation up. Practicing the "happy-dance" part of getting stuff done can help, even if you aren't the one who made the goal.

Just Be Better: Go watch local sports at a nearby park or field. Pick a side and really get into the game. It's best if you don't know anything about the teams or the sport for that matter. Keep cheering and do it liberally.

Enjoy in the accomplishment process and cheer like there's no tomorrow.

78) Just Browsing

There are two types of people when it comes to shopping: those that hate it and those that love it. Chances are, the people who hate it will just grumble or rush through the whole process as quickly as possible. On the other hand, those that love shopping will enjoy every last hour of shopping and sometimes without regard to costs.

I say don't be either type for a while. Instead, consider being the person that is inspired by shopping. Be someone who is intimately interested in the quality and construction of things out there. Inspect stuff and try to figure out how it was made. Picture the workers or machines that assembled the goods and get a feel for the whole manufacturing process.

Just Be Better: Go to a high-priced clothing, furniture, or electronics store. Browse, use, and gawk at the most awesome stuff you can find. Look for subtle features you wouldn't normally care about. Make it a point to not buy anything. Just observe and live it up.

Understand and appreciate the details of processes you take for granted.

79) If You Build It

There's something about the sandy part of going to the beach that's majestic. You've got tons of waves rolling in, minute upon minute, shaping the sand into a wonderful walkway. It adds just enough water and work to create a smooth surface and cool touch. If you stand there long enough, you can even feel the wet sand begin to hug your feet as you sink in. And do you know what the best part is? This sand is the ultimate stuff to make castles with.

Being surrounded by powerful forces all day and every day can make you feel out of control. Your boss, certain family members, mortgage companies, insurance agents, and even government officials can suck the feeling of self-control right out of you. It isn't until you can learn to shape the moldable pieces in life that their influence begins to have a lighter effect.

Just Be Better: Go to the beach and pick the nicest spot you can find. Feel the hot and powerful sun beat down on you, use and appreciate the massive waves crashing in, and gather the millions of pieces of sand around to make the best dang sandcastle ever. Experience and use the influence of the powerful forces around you to create something special. Take a picture of it. Now smash it to bits.

Have fun using the power around you to regain control of your life.

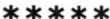

Be A Better Person:

BY COMMUNICATING

I don't think people realize how important their words are. Words are little packages of either good or bad being delivered to whoever is within earshot. And this includes you. The tongue truly is a mighty power that should be trained to be a powerful tool. And remember the permanency of things said on the internet. Let's start paying attention to what we say for everyone's benefit.

80) Stranger Smiles

As I was leaving Wal-Mart one day with my wife and kids, there were a couple of bored teens sitting around waiting for their parents to finish their shopping. I didn't know who they were but as we passed by, I let out a warm and friendly smile. Not those superficial, super-quick smiles you see at work, but an honest-to-goodness neighborly smile. Their faces lit up in an instant. From complete and utter boredom to almost a bright and sun-shiny happiness. It was a nice moment.

What can we say about little acts of kindness? Sure, there's a fine line between being a total creep and being a genuinely nice person. But you gain these skills with experience. If you don't bother to practice your "random acts of awesome-ness" skills, then you might stay in the "creep zone" for longer than you'd like. It's worth the effort to grow. A small gift of a smile can really brighten someone's day. This is a gift you can't place a value on.

Just Be Better: While you're out and about, compliment a stranger or acquaintance on their smile today. Don't be creepy. It helps if you start out with a small greeting first. Try something like, "Hi. I'm sitting here waiting for my kiddos to get situated and I just had to say I appreciate how well you're treating your kids. It's a good reminder for me. Enjoy your day!" Or maybe something along the lines of, "Hello. I'm just passing through, but I wanted to say you have an inspiring smile. Thanks for letting your personality shine. Bye!"

Be a minute-friend and spread the good cheer.

81) Turn that Frown Upside Down

Do you know someone who's especially good at pinpointing the faults in everything? Before any names or labels come to mind, it's a good time to stop thinking of that quality as a bad thing. Think of it as a skill they've acquired, but one that isn't always useful in every situation. Maybe you have this skill and are looking to add the other side of it to your toolbox? There's no reason to limit yourself to only one side.

There's research out there showing that in order for you to maintain a loving relationship with your family, you need to do at least five positive things for every one negative thing you do. That's the **positivity to negativity ratio** (P/N). Do I recommend keeping track of every single thing? No. Do I recommend making it a point to find opportunities to be positive and helpful? Yes. Turn your magnifying glass to what's done right, and be gentle with the mistakes.

http://en.wikipedia.org/wiki/Positivity/negativity_ratio

Just Be Better: Pay attention to what you say all day, whether it's out loud or in your head. Write down five negative things you say today. At the end of the day, scratch them out and write alternative, positive, and useful responses by each one. Use those new responses next time.

Accentuate the positive and grow your skills.

82) Boredom In Common

We go to great lengths to find the shortest line in the grocery store. Is it going to be the single guy with the bag of chips and a case of soda or the single mother with her three kids and a two-story tall shopping cart? There is an exact science to the process of finding the shortest line, as any experienced shopper will tell you. But is getting in and out always the best thing to do?

Much like texts and garage door openers, always trying to find the quickest way out is not good for building relationships. I'm not saying you need to make friends everywhere you go, but when's the last time you struck up a meaningful conversation with a stranger? The people you meet in life are some of the biggest influences to your personal growth and experience.

Just Be Better: Say hello and be genuinely interested in a stranger today while you wait. Try to get over the weather, politics, and talking about the long line. Look at something about them that hints at their interests. Let them talk about themselves.

Keep your opportunity door open and pick the long line every once in a while.

83) Naming Cashiers

I used to work at Albertsons in my early college days. Cutting meat and making cheesy announcements on the intercom was my gig. I was pretty good at it. You know what really threw me off track, but in a good way? When someone would come up and say, "Hey, Richard. Good to see you today." And the first thing through my mind was, "Whoa! How'd you know my name?!" As I look down and quickly remember my nametag.

A person's name is one of the most important triggers they've had since they were born. Think about it. From day one, their parents were using that one word to get their attention, show their love, and help them out. Over and over this one word was used as a signal for reaching into the kid's inner being. This is true for everyone.

Just Be Better: The next time you're out and about, preferably today, use the cashier's name while you're checking out. Wish them a good day, too. Try to talk about something other than work, if you can. End the checkout experience with a nice, "have a good day, Marty."

Treat names like gold and keep them polished with your attention.

84) Dog Gone It, People Like You

Think back to the last thing you did that you absolute, positively, horribly failed on. I'm talking about a complete and utterly embarrassing failure. What's the first thing that popped into your mind after it happened? Did you keep telling yourself something after that? Did anything you said to yourself help you recover from the mistake?

Most people default to being their own harshest critic. When something bad happens, some people have a bad habit of saying something like, "I'm so stupid!" or "I'll never get it right." or "I'm such a dork." Guess what? Your subconscious mind **doesn't know you're kidding**. Unknowingly, you're programming more failure into your being by saying meaningless things like that. Time for change.

http://psychology.uchicago.edu/people/faculty/cacioppo/jtcreprints/ilsc98.pdf

Just Be Better: Say five positive things to yourself today. Not to be all fluffy and stuff, but you really are a unique snowflake. There's no one else in the world just like you. You are as capable and intelligent as you try to be. You can say these positive things in your head, if you like. It certainly cuts back on the funky looks from others, if that matters anymore.

You've got to look at what you say to yourself to make changes you can grasp.

85) Two Ears, One Brain - Majority Wins

I could bore you with stories of how much trouble I've gotten into with my wife during our early days. Sure, things still pop up, but can you imagine the difficulty when she is trying to pour her thoughts out to me and I'm mentally keeping track of defenses to spit back at her instead of giving her my full attention. Thank God I've been taught some valuable lessons over the years.

Did you know the reason most people don't remember another person's name is because they weren't paying attention during the introduction? Can you imagine how little attention someone is paying when they're thinking about what to say while the other person is still talking? Communication is 7% words, 38% tone of voice, and 55% body language. You're missing out on 93% of the message if you think you're only ignoring the 7% you hear.

Just Be Better: Really listen, without thinking of what to say next, to at least three people today. Hear their words, notice how their tone of voice changes at different parts of the conversation, and look for big body shifts or changes in movement. These things are talking, too.

Communication is about digesting the whole picture, not just a quick glance.

86) 6 Second Pause

How do you feel when a telemarketer calls during your dinner and won't give up? You've said no seven times already and they keep pushing. I imagine your ability to care and be understanding goes down very quickly the longer the conversation gets. Granted, this is a situation not most people enjoy, but it does bring up a very important point about our default reactions.

Escalation is bringing something like emotions to a continually higher and higher level until a breaking point is reached. Escalation is such a horribly useless thing in a conversation, relationship, or negotiation. When emotions overcome any form of care, logic, or decency in an interaction, everyone loses. Our natural human reaction is to fight or flight in a confrontation. This isn't always useful in every situation. Learn to control this reaction and you'll notice huge changes in your life.

Just Be Better: The next time you're upset at someone, wait exactly six seconds before responding. Feel your face flush over, and try to make it stop. Literally count out six, five, four, three, two, one slowly in your head before you say anything. Keep practicing as it'll take some time to stick.

Take time to consider the cause by adding a pause.

*****

Be A Better Person:

BY CLEANING CHAOS

The clutter around us is a reflection of the clutter inside of us. The connection may be loose, but there's a reason for every bit of clutter around your house, in your car, and on your desk. By clearing the clutter, you can simultaneously work through why the junk made it there in the first place. Clear out your clutter and free your mind.

87) Chunk the Junk

From the day home builders starting putting in big basements, attics, and roomy garages, people have been finding ways to collect more stuff. Huge piles of empty boxes, appliances that were only used once, and exercise machines that were never taken out of their boxes. The extra spaces have become rooms to store the junk we don't want to deal with.

It's like those beliefs that held you back when you were a child. There were monsters under your bed, so you couldn't sleep or walk around at night, right? Every bit of clutter you have is a story waiting to be finished. Open stories are open loops in your mind. They take processing power away from you doing what matters.

Just Be Better: Get your resources back by chunking the junk in the garage, attic, and basement. No, you don't actually need the stuff. No, you won't get rich selling it on eBay. No, you won't need it in five years. No, your friends don't care about Christmas cards from thirteen years ago.

Close those old programs and reboot your machine, it's time to start fresh.

88) Junk in the Trunk

But what about those mobile homes we live in five days a week? What about our cars and trucks? We eat, shave, put on makeup, text, check Facebook, store trash, house books, hide papers and food scraps, and overall dump them full of the crumbs of our lives. Who cares about the back seat, right?

This is another one of those tell-tale life-junk areas. It's even worse than your home. Your home gets more attention from other folks that live there and has a better chance of being clean. But your personal mobile castle, your car, well, that's all you and only you. It can be a scary representation of the way you live life.

Just Be Better: Clean out all of the junk in your trunk. I'm talking about the car, people, the car. Organize what you can, and get rid of the rest of it. Don't worry about what other people think, but do think of what hints your "life-evidence" is saying about you.

What kind of story would a crime scene investigator tell about your life?

89) High Visibility

You know those super humid mornings during the rainy season? The ones where if you don't have your car's air conditioning system set just right, your windows fog over and make safe driving impossible. At that point, it's best to just pull over and clean every window and try again later.

Sometimes we need to clean our mental windows, our inner 'back-seat,' and our foggy minds. But where the heck does one start in that process? Properly taking care of the small things we often consider "out of sight, out of mind" will make that statement true: the problems will be solved and truly out of mind.

Just Be Better: Clean the back-seat of your car out. Do consider vacuuming. Wipe the back window with window-cleaner. Look at how dirty that rag is when you're done wiping. Did you know a rag could get so funky? Be amazed at how clear the view behind you is.

Layers of funk need a little attention – wipe on, wipe up, move on.

90) Gun the Bunnies

Your home is your castle. It keeps you warm, protects your privacy, and stores all of your goodies. Occasionally, you have to give it some tender love and care to get it ready for visitors or simply make a safe path to the bathroom.

Can cleaning your home be such a chore that only judgmental visitors give you the motivation to take action? This is usually because we care too much about what they think instead of what's ultimately good for us. You deserve cleanliness and orderliness no matter the company.

Just Be Better: Why not treat yourself as well as you would your visitors? Clean under your bed, cabinets, and in the corners. Get your dust-bunny gun ready as they don't like to be found.

You deserve higher standards. Keep your castle well taken care of.

91) Computing Dust

As the years go by, I think we're becoming more of a new type of technological creature. We use and rely on fancy machines to help answer and guide our actions. What once required a ruler, paper, pen, and a small miracle can now be done with laptops and smartphones in no time. Unless, of course, they don't work properly.

In some ways, technology can become a great crutch. A treasured device that solves your problem in under a second can become a nightmare when it goes wonky. It isn't until our tools of convenience go bad that we realize how much we rely on them.

Just Be Better: Clean the outside of your computer and smartphones. Vacuum the dust and hairballs out of the vents and cracks. Wipe the keyboard, mouse, and screen with a cloth, not water. Keep those tools in top working order.

Technology moves fast and breaks faster. Maintain your sanity and don't take it for granted.

92) Naked No More

I grew up sharing everything from shoes, to pants, to hole-filled socks with my two brothers. We weren't the richest bunch in the neighborhood and had to cut some corners. But you know what made us feel better? Getting that new (to us) hand-me-down because we had something to call our own. Plus, it felt nice to share the stuff I didn't need with those dorky dudes.

A sense of ownership is one of the basic human needs. Similarly, the sense of worth and value gained by being able to help others hits the higher-level human needs. It isn't until you have the lower-level need filled that you can finally start focusing on the higher-level stuff.

Just Be Better: Go through and donate clothes you no longer need. Do the higher-level thing and clothe the naked and needy. Your local charities will be glad to take it all or there are usually drop boxes in large store parking lots.

Help those in need to help themselves, one level at a time.

93) Clear a Path

I love my family to no end and though it doesn't happen enough, I enjoy traveling to see them in their far off places. The older and wiser folks in the family tree aren't as spry as they used to be and could use an extra hand sometimes. I'm a big supporter of the "take care of your own" mindset and it makes for an even more fulfilling trip.

It's easy to feel forgotten when we're not close to the outside world and those who love us most. The mature generation does matter a great deal and has so much to contribute to your life and the entire world. Tap into those great folks in your family tree.

Just Be Better: Plan your next trip to the least-visited grandparents. Make it a big deal and have a good time. Offer to do, and follow through, at least three big chores that need to get done and have the biggest impact on their lives.

A maturing love is a fine candidate for extra giving. Own up and give back.

94) A Book is a Terrible Thing to Waste

I don't know what I'd do without books. I don't care if they're paper, digital, broken, long, short, whatever, as long as they have at least one little nugget of awesome information inside. I know it's there and I will find it. And then it's time to share it with the world.

It's been said that the biggest difference between a successful person and a failure is the people they've met and the books they've read. Read, read, and read some more. Then it's time to put your learning to good use for yourself and for others. And share your story with others, too.

Just Be Better: Finish up that self-help book, that gripping novel, and that biography. It's time to sift through and donate books you are done with. Goodwill needs them now.

Be the knowledge then share the gift.

*****

Be A Better Person:

IN SOCIETY

We weren't made to keep everything to ourselves. We're a people built on community, sharing, and helping each other out. The more we learn to love the world, the more we begin to see we need to give back. Share your time, talents, and treasure with the world. It'll share back and it'll grow with you.

95) I Like What You Did There

You know what brings a smile to my son's face when he's doing a project or building with his building blocks? A small, totally unnecessary, but absolutely genuine compliment on the way he's doing what he's doing. There's something about the random comment from good-old-loving daddy that seems to make things that much more special.

Humans don't like labels. Sure, labels make things easier to work with but they also make things easier to dismiss. They're also horrible for learning, motivation, and growing overall. But, if we can start focusing more on the 'how' we do things instead of the 'what,' then we can begin to build from the inside.

Just Be Better: Whether you're at work, home, or the store, appreciate the work of someone else today. Be kind, be genuine, and make it count. Say something that will stick with them forever. Make a good movement happen.

Take note of the awesome in others and share it with them.

96) A Bag of Kindness

I'm amazed at the kind people that came out of the woodworks to give us tons of wonderful clothes when our baby boy and girl were born. And these clothes aren't cheap, let me tell you. Talk about a wonderful feeling knowing we weren't only cared for but we could now show extra care for our lovely new additions.

A comfortable world can be simultaneously awesome and saddening. So many people go without necessities while so many other people have so much. Yet, many people with much on the outside are missing even more on the inside. Well, here's a secret to those with a surplus of resources. Here's a great way to help build you up from the inside. Those lovely people around you could use your help.

Just Be Better: Donate a grocery bag's worth of canned goods to your local charity or church. It doesn't matter what you bring, but it'd be mighty nice if you called ahead and asked what they needed. Buy extra. Repeat often.

Canning the Grinch and helping the needy is a cinch.

97) Teach a Man to Fish

Ever had a buddy bug you for a few bucks? Did you expect to get it back? I mean, who cares, right? It's only a few bucks and you're pals. If you can be out a few dollars you won't miss anyway, it's worth it to help someone special to you. Of course, you'd like to think he was using it for a good cause, but that never comes up. But what if it did?

Sometimes we get in a habit of not really caring what happens to the good we do in life. It becomes second-nature and we miss a little of the importance of our actions in the happenings of the day. What if you could start giving gifts that directly changed people's lives? I'm talking a 180 degree turn, from the ground up, revolutionary change for a couple of bucks.

Micro-financing is an awesome program where you can loan as little as twenty-five dollars to entrepreneurs in developing countries. It enables them to buy farm equipment, fertilizer for crops, and more. The program has an over 98% payback rate. It's absolutely amazing.

Just Be Better: Go over to **Kiva's website** and lend a few bucks to a Kiva entrepreneur. You'll get it back and help someone in the process. You might even make a family friend and change a small community for life.

http://www.kiva.org/start

This is permanent change, from your pocket change. You dig?

98) Reach Out And Help Someone

I remember stumbling across my church's website one day and thinking to myself, "wow, this needs some serious work." Mass times were wrong, directions were missing, and it was overall a lackluster experience. Well, I figured there's no time like now to offer my free help. They were ecstatic and there's no telling how many people it helped. Talk about a heart-lifter.

I didn't just give them money and point them to a website developer. I rolled up my sleeves and got to work. Don't get me wrong, every charity is looking for more resources to help run their operations. But sometimes the most important resource is people. All the money in the world won't help a humanitarian effort if there's no one to do the work.

Just Be Better: Research a charity or church in your area to see if they could use a hand every once in a while. Offer to help them with your time, talent, or treasures. Start with your time.

Use some of your time to do the good Lord's work. The world needs you.

99) Part the Clouds

Don't get me started on those super-grumpy, no-coffee-yet Mondays. Yeah I'm a little more cheery than most folks and I may still have a smile on my face, but sometimes it's an absolute battle to keep it going in the middle of a busy day. But it's what we do to keep going. If we don't do it, who will?

There are plenty of people out there that can't cope as well as most folks. We can help them out by lending a little of our cheer and appreciation their way. And even better than that, sometimes the best gift is to be more patient when you're sensing someone is having a bad day. A little understanding on your part goes a long way.

Just Be Better: Give a word of encouragement to someone having a bad day. A smile will work, too. Give them extra space when they show their Monday-morning fangs. We're people first, coworkers second.

Share your good cheer - it's contagious.

100) A Beautiful Day in the Neighborhood

How many times do you stand in the driveway and talk to your neighbors as they come home from a long day's work? Do you know your neighbor's names? Or do you hit the automatic garage door opener, speed in, and let the door fall back down as quickly as it went up? I've been guilty of this a few times too many. Hey, I'm learning, too.

Our homes are our castles. We do all we do there and they are the foundations of our comfort, safety, and the expression of who we are. So why don't we pay more attention to the people and things surrounding our fortress? Are we letting the weeds weaken our foundation? Are we missing great opportunities to combine forces and grow? We'll never know until we know.

Just Be Better: Offer to help a neighbor with the yard, house maintenance, or babysitting. Do it for free. You're trying to build on a great foundation here. Do it right and do it like you mean it.

Be a good neighbor and build the community.

101) Rewarding Progress

I helped run a cookie contest at one of my corporate jobs. It was a lot of fun and we gave away some great prizes. But you know what seemed to make the biggest impact? The little "You're a Winner" certificates I made for first and second place were a huge hit. The second place winner had long since spent her fifty dollar prize, but one year later she still had her certificate up on her cube wall.

Words work wonders as you're probably finding out. But sometimes they don't have the same meaning as a tangible object. Something we can look over, touch, feel, and be a part of. There's a reason people give trophies and flowers instead of pats on the back and little smooches. Doing one type of reward is great, but doing both is absolutely fantastic.

Just Be Better: Let's start at home as they're the folks that need our biggest and best rewards of love the most. Recognize an accomplishment of a family member. Make a handmade award for the younger ones. Make it grand, make it special, and make it permanent.

Give a tangible exchange and make a difference in someone's heart.

*****

Well on Your Way to Being a Better You

Congratulations on making it through all 101 ways to help make you a better person. That's a lot of good work and you should celebrate your successes. Whether it's been a one-percent change or a complete redo, thank you for committing yourself to growing yourself.

I had a lot of fun doing these exercises myself as well as writing this book. I really do believe this book will help you grow, if it hasn't already.

Thank you for being a better person, thank you for helping the world be better, and thank you for being better in the future. Keep on growing and remember to check back when you're looking for ideas.

And most important of all...

Forget Perfect, Just Be Better.

*****

About Richard N. Stephenson

I'm the elbow-grease behind RichardStep: Self-Assessment Tools for the Entrepreneur in You (**http://richardstep.com**), helping thousands discover more about themselves daily. I've published several books on personality testing, optimizing learning, and building strengths. I've also designed online self-discovery, strengths, and motivation tests on richardstep.com.

Cancer once knocked me down, the good Lord gave me a second chance, and now I want to help you use yours. I take the old personal development fluff and turn it into tools you can use. My latest tool, Unleash Your Strengths (**http://getuys.com**), is guaranteed to help you in your journey.

I live near Houston, TX, with my extraordinary wife, adorable kids, and overgrown backyard.

Please feel free to contact me. I'm always looking for more life enhancing hints and tips.

AMAZON:
http://amazon.com/author/richardnstephenson
EMAIL: **mailto:richard@richardstep.com**
TWITTER: **http://twitter.com/rstephenson_**
VIDEOS: **http://youtube.com/rstephensonable**
ADDRESS:
PO Box 3395
League City, TX, 77574-3395

Other Books by Richard N. Stephenson

See my **Amazon Author page** for my latest books on
Amazon - http://bit.ly/rnsamazon

See my **blog author page** for my latest books overall -
http://richardstep.com/products/

Be Your Own Life Coach Series:

* Vol. 1: Learning to Learn More
* Vol. 2: How to Find Your Passion & Purpose in Life

Self-Discovery Series:

* Jungian 16 Types Personality Test
* DOPE 4 Bird Personality Test
* Unleash Your Strengths: Take the Test & Guide Your
Change

Other Titles:

* 435 Simple YouTube Video Ideas and Movie Making
Tips

One Last Thing

When you turn the page, you'll get the opportunity to rate this book and share a two or three sentence review of your experience here.

If you believe this book is worth reading, would you take a few seconds to let your friends know about it? If it turns out to make a difference in their lives, they'll be grateful to you. As I will.

I'm an independent publisher and your review means a lot to other people considering this investment. It really does help when you share your thoughts and feelings.

Thank you,
Richard N. Stephenson

PS) If you'd rather share your thoughts directly on Amazon, the book's link is here:

http://www.amazon.com/Richard-N.-
Stephenson/e/B006BJ0QA8

www.ingramcontent.com/pod-product-compliance
Lightning Source LLC
Chambersburg PA
CBHW070120290526
45789CB00005B/2084